THE ULTIMATE DIVERTICULITIS HANDBOOK

Your Essential Guide to Understanding and Managing Flare-Ups.

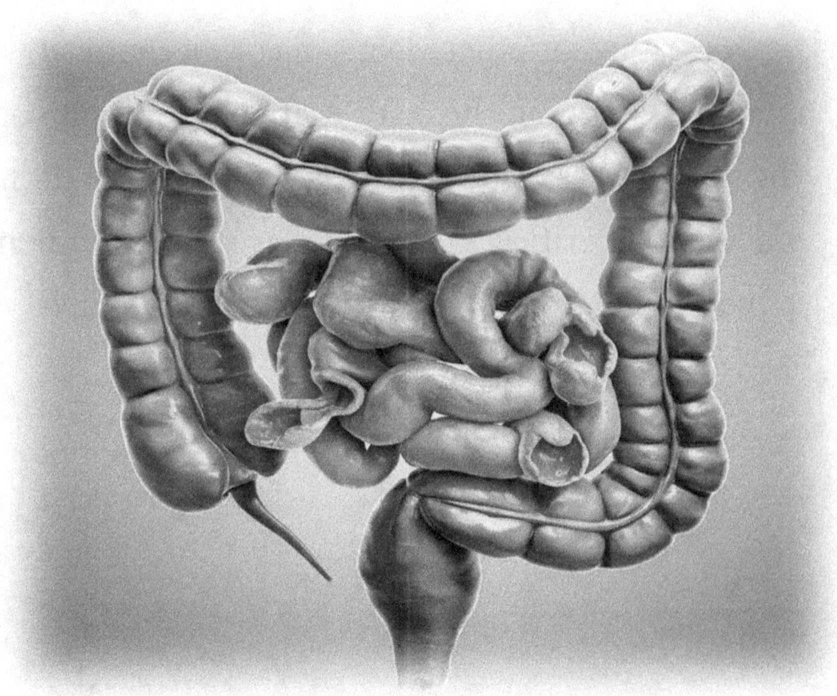

CHRISTIANA WHITE

Craving Delicious Meals That Also Support Your Gut Health?

We've got you covered! Scan this QR code to discover our collection of Diverticulitis Cookbooks:

- **Diverticulitis Diet Cookbook**: Flavorful recipes to nourish your body and prevent flare-ups
- **Diverticulitis Diet Cookbook for Seniors**: Tailored meals for older adults managing diverticulitis
- **Diverticulitis Smoothies Recipes**: Quick & easy nutrient-packed smoothies to soothe your gut

Scan now and start your journey to delicious, gut-friendly eating!

TABLE OF CONTENTS.

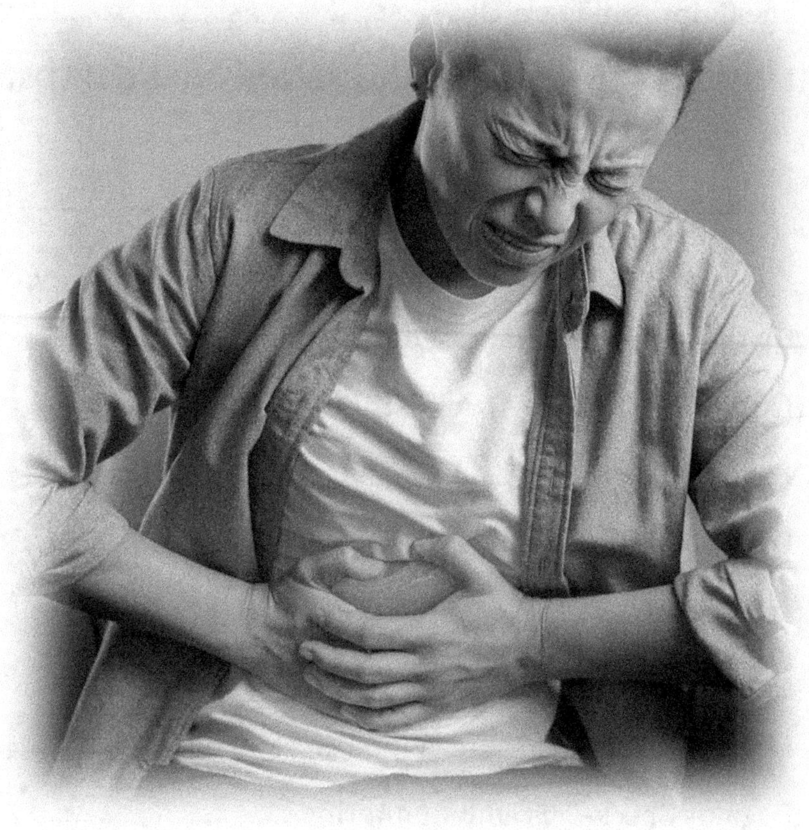

INTRODUCTION

Imagine a life in which the fear of unexpected, terrible abdominal pain no longer influences your decisions. Imagine yourself eating meals without tension, traveling without concern, and seizing every opportunity with confidence. This is the life that awaits you outside of diverticulitis flare-ups.

Countless people have previously recognized the transformational potential of information and proactive management. They've learned to understand their bodies' subtle signals, negotiate the complexities of treatment options, and adopt lifestyle modifications that promote long-term well-being. Their stories demonstrate the resiliency of the human spirit and the powerful influence of enlightened self-care.

Within these pages, you'll discover a wealth of ideas, methods, and practical guidance, all thoughtfully prepared to help you on your own path to digestive independence. Whether you've recently been diagnosed, want to learn more about your disease, or want to avoid future flare-ups, this handbook is a reliable resource.

We'll demystify the complexities of diverticulitis, look into its causes and triggers, and give you the tools you need to properly manage flare-ups. We'll look at the most recent research on dietary and lifestyle changes, providing evidence-based advice to improve your gut health and reduce the risk of problems.

However, this is not just a guide. It's an invitation to reclaim your life, to take a proactive approach to your health, and to develop a sense of empowerment in the face of a difficult disease.

"The Ultimate Diverticulitis Handbook" is your key to a future in which you not just manage but thrive after diverticulitis. Let's take this trip together, one step at a time, to a life of increased comfort, confidence, and well-being.

CHAPTER ONE: UNDERSTANDING DIVERTICULITIS

What Is Diverticulitis?

Definition and Prevalence

Diverticulitis is a disorder characterized by the inflammation or infection of tiny pouches called diverticula that can form in the digestive tract's walls, particularly in the colon. These pouches form when weak places in the colon wall give way under strain, allowing parts to protrude out. Diverticula are usually innocuous and asymptomatic, but when they become inflamed or infected, they create diverticulitis, which can cause substantial discomfort gastrointestinal difficulties.

Diverticulitis is quite frequent, particularly in Western countries. Diverticulosis, or the presence of diverticula, is believed to affect approximately 35% of the Western world's population.

Approximately 4-15% of people with diverticulosis may develop diverticulitis. Diverticulosis becomes increasingly common with age, affecting more than 30% of those aged 50 to 59 and over 70% of those aged 80 and older.

Diverticulosis vs. Diverticulitis

Diverticulosis and diverticulitis are similar but separate conditions:

• **Diverticulosis**: This term refers to the presence of diverticula in the colon. It is frequently asymptomatic and is detected coincidentally during routine screens or imaging exams.

Diverticulosis does not create symptoms and does not require treatment beyond dietary changes to avoid complications.

• **Diverticulitis**: This condition develops when one or more diverticula become inflamed or infected. Diverticulitis symptoms include severe abdominal discomfort, fever, nausea, and changes in bowel habits including constipation or diarrhea.

Unlike diverticulosis, diverticulitis necessitates medical treatment, which may include antibiotics, dietary adjustments, and, in severe cases, surgery.

Risk Factors and Lifestyle Influences

Several risk factors and lifestyle effects might raise the risk of getting diverticulitis:

- Age: The risk of diverticulitis rises with age, especially after age 50.
- Diet: A diet low in fiber and high in red meat is linked to an increased incidence of diverticulitis. Fiber softens feces and reduces intestinal pressure, potentially preventing the formation of diverticula.
- Obesity: Being overweight or obese raises your risk of diverticulitis.
- Physical inactivity: A sedentary lifestyle has been related to an increased risk of diverticulitis. Regular physical activity promotes bowel regularity and reduces colon pressure.
- Smoking: This is a proven risk factor for diverticulitis.
- Medications: Certain medications, including nonsteroidal anti-inflammatory drugs (NSAIDs), steroids, and opioids, can raise the risk of diverticulitis.
- Genetics: Having a family history of diverticulitis increases a person's susceptibility.

Understanding these risk factors is critical for taking preventive steps and lowering your chances of developing diverticulitis flare-ups.

Lifestyle changes, notably following a high-fiber diet and engaging in regular physical activity, can help manage and avoid this illness.

Anatomy of Digestive System

An Overview of The Digestive Tract.

The digestive system is a complicated network of organs that breaks down food, absorbs nutrients, and eliminates waste. It is made up of several main components:

- Mouth: The first stage of digestion, where food is chewed and combined with saliva.
- Esophagus: A muscular tube that moves food from the mouth to the stomach.
- Stomach: A sac-like organ that further digests food with acids and enzymes.
- The small intestine is the principal site of nutrition absorption.

- The large intestine (colon) is responsible for absorbing water and storing waste before elimination.
- Rectum and Anus: The final stages of the digestive tract, when waste is evacuated from the body.

Each portion of the digestive tract is essential to the overall digesting process. However, diverticulitis primarily affects the large intestine.

Large Intestine and Diverticula Formation

The large intestine, often known as the colon, is the last segment of the digestive tract.

It is around 5 feet long and larger in diameter than the small intestine. The colon's principal roles are:

- Water absorption: The colon collects water from the remaining food, which solidifies into stool.
- Waste storage: Stool is kept in the colon until it is removed by the body.
- Vitamin production: Bacteria in the colon contribute to the production of some vitamins, including vitamin K.

Diverticula Formation.

Diverticula are tiny pouches that can expand through weak places in the colon wall. They are most typically found in the sigmoid colon, which is the S-shaped section of the colon closest to the rectum.

The specific reason of diverticula formation is unknown, but it is thought to be due to increased pressure within the colon. This pressure can occur when the colon muscles work harder to move stool, especially if the stool is hard and dry as a result of a low-fiber diet.

Over time, this increased pressure can cause the inner layers of the colon wall to push through weak points in the outer muscle layers, resulting in diverticula.

Key Points:

- Diverticula are most commonly found in the sigmoid colon.
- A low-fiber diet is a significant risk factor for diverticulum formation.
- Diverticula are usually innocuous (diverticulosis).
- However, they may become inflamed or infected, resulting in diverticulitis.

Understanding the anatomy of the large intestine and the process of diverticula formation lays the groundwork for understanding how diverticulitis occurs and how it can be controlled and prevented.

The Culprits of Flare-Ups

Inflammation and Infection: Underlying Mechanisms

The exact trigger for this process is not always evident, although it is suspected to entail a mix of factors:

- **Obstruction**: A little piece of stool or undigested food can become stuck in a diverticulum and cause a blockage. This blockage can cause bacterial overgrowth and irritation.
- **Microperforation**: The trapped material can create a tiny tear or perforation in the diverticulum wall, allowing germs to escape into the surrounding tissues and cause an infection.
- **Immune Response:** The body's immune system reacts to the inflammation or infection, causing further swelling, discomfort, and other symptoms.

Diverticulitis-related inflammation and infection might be moderate or severe. In moderate situations, the inflammation may resolve itself with conservative treatment.

In more severe cases, problems such as abscess formation, perforation, or peritonitis (inflammation of the abdominal lining) may ensue.

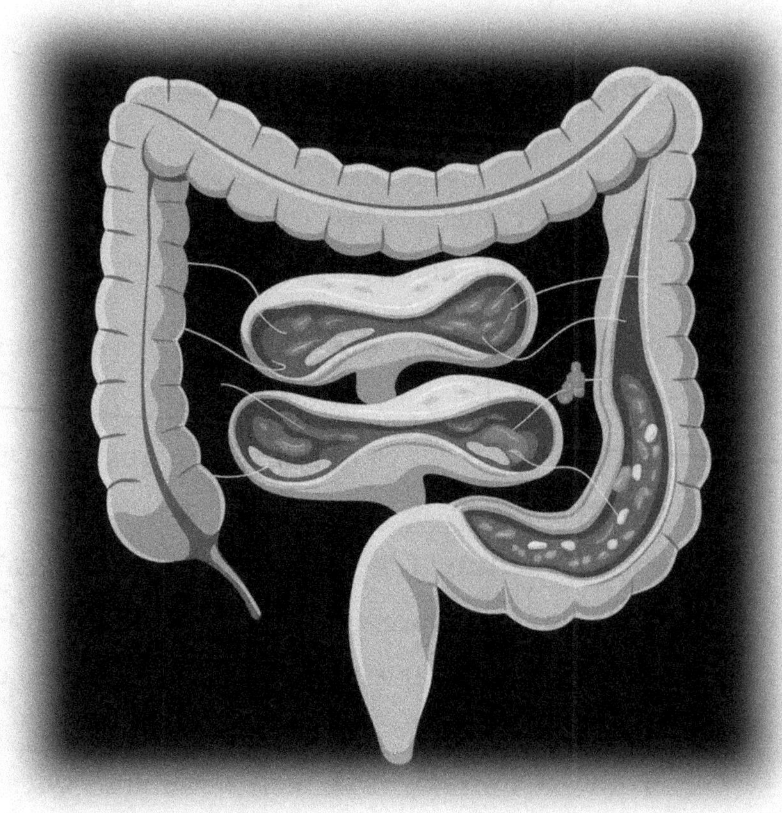

CHAPTER TWO: RECOGNIZING SIGNS AND SYMPTOMS

Common Symptoms of a Flare-Up

A diverticulitis flare-up can present with a wide range of symptoms, from minor discomfort to severe pain and consequences.

Recognizing these signs early is critical for receiving proper medical assistance and avoiding severe issues.

Abdominal Pain's Characteristics

Abdominal discomfort is the most prevalent and visible sign of a diverticulitis flare-up. Pain is typically:

- The sigmoid colon, which is the most common site of diverticula, is located in the lower left abdomen. However, discomfort can also be felt in other parts of the abdomen.
- Persistent and crampy: The discomfort is commonly described as a dull aching with occasional severe cramps.

- Worsens with movement or pressure: Coughing, sneezing, or even walking might aggravate the pain.
- Passing gas or having a bowel movement might temporarily reduce pressure in the colon.

The pain might range from minor discomfort to acute anguish.

If you have sudden, severe stomach discomfort, particularly if it is accompanied by other symptoms such as fever or vomiting, seek medical assistance right once.

Changes In Bowel Habits

Diverticulitis can affect normal bowel movement, resulting in a variety of bowel habits:

- Constipation: This is a frequent complaint caused by inflammation and constriction of the colon.
- Diarrhea: In some circumstances, diverticulitis can produce diarrhea, especially if there is an infection.
- Alternating constipation and diarrhea: This might happen as the problem worsens.
- Blood in stool: While not always present, blood in the stool may indicate bleeding from an inflamed or

diseased diverticulum. This requires an immediate medical assessment.

Any major or persistent changes in bowel habits should be reported to your doctor, as they may suggest a flare-up or another underlying digestive problem.

Nausea, Vomiting, And Fever.

These symptoms frequently accompany a diverticulitis flare-up, especially if there is severe inflammation or infection.

- Nausea and vomiting: These symptoms are caused by inflammation and irritation in the digestive tract.
- Fever: A fever indicates that the body is fighting an infection. It is frequently accompanied by chills and general malaise.

If you have persistent nausea, vomiting, or fever, seek medical help right away, as these symptoms may signal a dangerous infection that requires immediate treatment.

Other Potential Symptoms

In addition to the preceding, diverticulitis flare-ups can cause:

- Bloating and gas: These symptoms may be caused by changes in intestinal function or bacterial overgrowth.
- Loss of appetite: This is frequently accompanied by nausea and abdominal pain.
- Fatigue and weakness: These symptoms may be caused by the body's efforts to combat infection and inflammation.
- Urinary symptoms: In some situations, diverticulitis can irritate the bladder, causing frequent urination or a burning feeling when urinating.

While these symptoms are not as common as the principal ones stated above, they can nevertheless cause discomfort and a lower quality of life during a flare up.

Remember to see your doctor if you notice any of these symptoms, especially if they are severe or persistent.

Early diagnosis and treatment are critical for successfully controlling diverticulitis and avoiding complications.

<u>When to Seek Medical Attention?</u>

While some diverticulitis flare-ups are small and heal with cautious home therapy, others progress quickly and result in significant consequences.

Recognizing the warning signals and seeking medical help as soon as possible is critical for accurate diagnosis and treatment.

Red Flags and Warning Signs

If you have any of the following symptoms, you should seek emergency medical assistance.

- Severe abdominal pain: Pain that is strong, persistent, or intensifies with time.
- High fever: A persistent or recurrent fever above 101°F (38.3°C).
- Chills and shaking may accompany a high fever and signal a dangerous infection.
- Bloody stools: Blood in your stool, whether brilliant red or black and sticky, requires rapid attention.
- Persistent nausea and vomiting: Inability to consume water or food might result in dehydration and electrolyte abnormalities.

- Signs of intestinal obstruction include severe constipation, inability to pass gas, and abdominal distention (bloating).
- Signs of peritonitis include severe stomach pain, soreness, stiffness, fever, and a fast heart rate. Peritonitis is a medical emergency that requires rapid surgical treatment.

The Value of Early Diagnosis and Treatment

Early detection and treatment of diverticulitis is critical for various reasons:

- **Complication prevention**: Early therapy can help prevent the inflammation and infection from progressing, lowering the risk of consequences like abscess formation, perforation, peritonitis, and sepsis.
- **Reducing discomfort and pain:** Prompt medical attention can relieve symptoms and enhance quality of life during a flare-up.
- **Reducing the need for surgery**: Early treatment with antibiotics and other conservative methods can often prevent surgical intervention.
- **Improving long-term outcomes**: By responding quickly to flare-ups and adopting required lifestyle

changes, you can lessen the frequency and severity of future episodes while also improving your overall digestive health.

Diagnostic Tools and Procedures.

An accurate diagnosis is critical for properly controlling and treating diverticulitis.

Healthcare experts use a combination of clinical assessments and diagnostic testing to establish the presence of diverticulitis and determine its severity.

Physical Exam and Medical History

The diagnosis process usually starts with a comprehensive physical exam and a review of your medical history. The doctor will:

- Evaluate your symptoms: They will ask about the type, location, length, and severity of your stomach pain, as well as any other symptoms you may be experiencing.
- Perform a physical examination, which will include palpating your abdomen for pain, guarding, or lumps.

- Review your medical history: They will inquire about your previous medical issues, surgeries, medications, and family history of diverticular disease.

This initial screening assists your doctor in determining the likelihood of diverticulitis and guiding subsequent diagnostic testing.

Imaging Tests

Imaging examinations are critical for verifying and measuring the severity of diverticulitis.

- **CT scan**: A computed tomography (CT) scan is the most common imaging test used to diagnose diverticulitis. It captures precise images of the belly and pelvis, allowing your doctor to see the colon, identify inflammatory diverticula, and discover problems such abscesses or perforations.
- **Ultrasound**: An ultrasound may be utilized in some circumstances, especially if there is a risk of complications such an abscess. However, it is less sensitive than a CT scan in detecting diverticulitis.
- **X-ray**: An abdominal X-ray can be used to rule out other causes of abdominal discomfort, such as bowel

blockage or perforation, but it is not specific for detecting diverticulitis.

Blood Tests and Stool Samples

- **Blood tests**: A complete blood count (CBC) can detect indicators of illness, such as an increase in white blood cell counts. Other blood tests, such as CRP and ESR, can also detect inflammation.
- **Stool samples**: A stool sample may be tested for blood, which could indicate bleeding from an inflamed diverticulum. Stool cultures can also be used to determine the exact bacteria causing the ailment.

Colonoscopy

A colonoscopy is a technique that involves introducing a flexible tube containing a camera into the rectum to view the whole colon.

It is usually avoided during an acute diverticulitis flare-up due to the danger of perforation. However, it may be advised when the irritation has decreased to:

- Confirm the diagnosis: A colonoscopy can assist visualize diverticula and determine the level of inflammation or scarring.

- Rule out other conditions: This can help rule out other possible reasons of your symptoms, such as colorectal cancer or inflammatory bowel disease.

- Determine the necessity for surgery: In some circumstances, a colonoscopy may be utilized to assess the severity of the condition and if surgery is required.

Your doctor's recommendations for diagnostic testing will be based on your personal circumstances and the severity of your symptoms.

If you have any questions or concerns concerning the diagnostic process, please discuss them with your healthcare professional.

They will be able to explain the reasoning behind each test and what to expect.

CHAPTER THREE: MANAGING FLARE-UPS

Treatment Options

The treatment for diverticulitis is determined by the intensity of the flare-up, the existence of comorbidities, and your overall health.

It might range from cautious home care to hospitalization and surgical intervention.

Conservative Management

Conservative home treatment may be adequate for mild instances of diverticulitis without consequences. This often includes:

- Rest: Getting enough rest allows your body to focus on healing and combating inflammation.
- Dietary Changes: Initially, a clear liquid diet may be recommended to rest your bowels. As your symptoms improve, gradually reintroduce low-fiber foods and finally return to a high-fiber diet.
- Antibiotics: Oral antibiotics are frequently administered to treat the infection caused by

diverticulitis. The type and duration of antibiotics will be determined by the severity of your ailment and any underlying health conditions.

- Discomfort Management: For mild to moderate discomfort, over-the-counter pain medications such acetaminophen (Tylenol) may be advised. If necessary, your doctor may prescribe stronger painkillers.

Pain Management

Managing discomfort is a vital part of diverticulitis treatment. In addition to over-the-counter pain medicines, your doctor could prescribe:

- Prescription pain pills: If over-the-counter medications do not work, your doctor may prescribe stronger pain relievers, such as opioids, for short-term usage.
- Antispasmodics: These drugs can relax the muscles of the colon, reducing cramps and pain.

To avoid potential adverse effects and reliance, you should strictly adhere to your doctor's directions for pain medication dosage and duration.

Hospitalization

Hospitalization could be necessary if:

- You have severe symptoms, such as a high temperature, continuous vomiting, or evidence of intestinal obstruction or peritonitis.
- You cannot tolerate oral intake: If you are unable to drink fluids or take medications owing to nausea and vomiting, you may require intravenous fluids and medications in a hospital setting.
- You have problems including an abscess, perforation, or fistula (an improper connection between the colon and another organ).
- You have other underlying health concerns, which may complicate your recovery or raise the chance of complications.

You will be closely watched while in the hospital, given intravenous fluids and antibiotics, and may have additional tests or procedures performed, such as a CT scan or abscess drainage.

Surgical Interventions

Surgery may be recommended in several instances, including:

- Recurrent diverticulitis: If you have repeated flare-ups despite conservative treatment.
- Complications: abscess, perforation, fistula, or stricture (colon narrowing).
- Uncontrolled bleeding: In rare circumstances, diverticulitis can produce severe bleeding necessitating surgical intervention.

There are various surgical techniques for diverticulitis, including:

- Primary bowel resection: This procedure removes the diseased portion of the colon and reconnects the healthy ends.
- Laparoscopic surgery: This minimally invasive procedure employs small incisions and specialized devices, generally resulting in quicker recovery times.
- Colonoscopy combined with endoscopic operations: In some circumstances, less invasive endoscopic techniques might be performed to drain an abscess or treat a fistula.

The sort of surgery recommended will be based on your personal circumstances and the severity of the sickness.

Dietary Strategies for a Flare Up

Dietary changes are critical for controlling diverticulitis flare-ups. The main goals of dietary changes during an episode are to:

- Rest the bowel: Allowing your digestive system to rest can help reduce inflammation and improve healing.
- Reduce irritation: Avoid foods that may cause or worsen symptoms.
- Stay hydrated: Maintain fluid intake to avoid dehydration and improve overall health.

Clear Liquid Diet

During the early phases of a flare-up, when symptoms are most intense, your doctor may recommend a clear liquid diet.

This diet comprises of easily digestible fluids that leave little residue in the digestive tract. Examples of transparent liquids are:

- Water.
- Clear broth or bouillon.
- Clear fruit juices (no pulp)
- Gelatin
- Popsicles.
- Tea or coffee (no milk or cream).

The clear liquid diet is usually followed for a few days, or until your symptoms begin to improve.

It is critical to avoid solid foods and dairy products during this stage.

Gradual Reintroduction of Foods

As your symptoms improve, you can gradually reintroduce items into your diet. Begin with low-fiber, easily digested foods, such as:

- Cooked veggies without skins or seeds.
- Ripe bananas.
- Apple sauce.
- White rice.
- Plain Yogurt
- Scrambled eggs.

Gradually increase the quantity and variety of meals as tolerated, eventually returning to a high-fiber diet.

This gradual approach helps to avoid overwhelming your digestive system and reduces the danger of causing more inflammation.

Foods to Avoid.

During a diverticulitis flare-up, it is critical to avoid foods that irritate the digestive tract or exacerbate symptoms. This includes:

- High-fiber meals: While a high-fiber diet can help with long-term management, it is better to avoid high-fiber foods during a flare-up since they can increase bowel movement and perhaps worsen inflammation. Examples include raw fruits and vegetables, entire grains, nuts, and seeds.
- Spicy Foods: They might irritate the digestive tract and worsen symptoms.
- Fatty or fried foods are difficult to digest and may cause nausea and diarrhea.
- Alcohol and caffeine can irritate the intestines and exacerbate symptoms.
- Carbonated beverages: They can induce bloating and gas, which can be unpleasant during a flare-up.

Staying hydrated is critical during a diverticulitis flare-up, especially if you're having diarrhea or vomiting.

Adequate fluid consumption reduces dehydration, softens stools, and promotes general recovery. Aim to consume plenty of water and other clear drinks throughout the day.

Remember:

- Follow your doctor's precise dietary recommendations, which may differ depending on the severity of your flare-up and any other underlying health concerns.
- Pay attention to your body and avoid any foods that appear to provoke or exacerbate your symptoms.
- If you have any questions or concerns about your nutrition during a flare-up, contact your doctor or a certified dietitian. They can offer personalized advice and support.

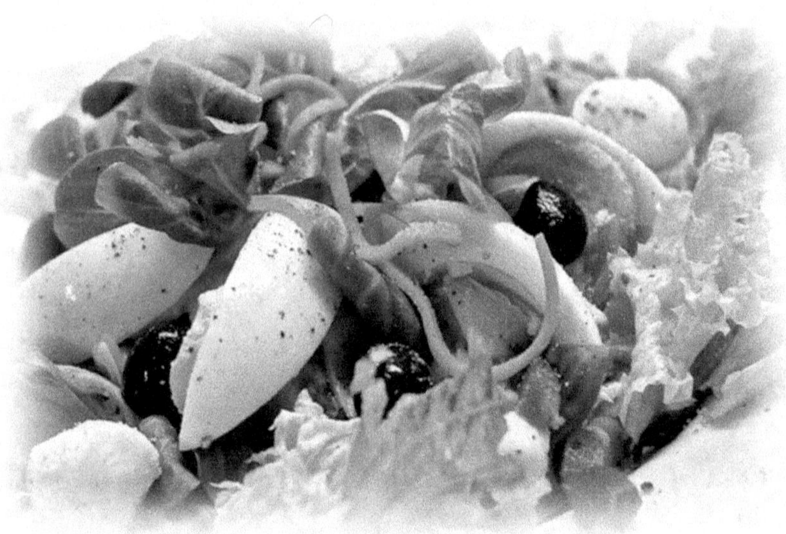

CHAPTER FOUR: PREVENTING FUTURE FLARE-UPS

Dietary Guidelines for Long-Term Management

After a diverticulitis flare-up has passed and you've returned to a regular diet, implementing a long-term dietary approach centered on gut health can dramatically minimize the risk of future episodes and boost overall digestive well-being.

High Fiber Diet

A high-fiber diet is regarded as the cornerstone of diverticulitis prevention. Fiber bulks up the stool, making it easier to pass and relieving strain on the colon.

This can assist to prevent the production of new diverticula and reduce the risk of existing ones becoming inflamed or infected.

The recommended daily fiber intake for adults is:

- Men: 38 grams.
- Women: 25 grams.

However, to minimize gas and bloating, increase your fiber intake gradually. Begin by adding a few grams of fiber per day, gradually working your way up to the suggested level.

Fiber-Rich Foods

Include a wide range of fiber-rich foods in your diet, including:

- Fruits: strawberries, apples, pears, bananas, and oranges.
- Vegetables include broccoli, Brussels sprouts, carrots, spinach, and kale.
- Whole grains include brown rice, quinoa, oats, whole wheat bread, and whole wheat pasta.
- Legumes include lentils, beans, chickpeas, and peas.
- Nuts and seeds include almonds, walnuts, chia seeds, and flaxseeds.

Whole foods are preferable to processed foods because they contain more fiber and other critical elements.

Probiotics And Prebiotics.

- Probiotics: These are live helpful bacteria that can help to maintain a healthy gut flora. They are present in fermented foods such as yogurt, kefir, sauerkraut, and kimchi, as well as probiotic supplements.
- Prebiotics: These are non-digestible fibers that provide sustenance for the good bacteria in your stomach. They can be found in foods such as onions, garlic, bananas, asparagus, and whole grains.

Including both probiotics and prebiotics in your diet can help sustain a healthy gut microbiota, perhaps lowering your risk of diverticulitis flare-ups.

Supplements

While a healthy diet should give the majority of the nutrients you require, some persons with diverticulitis may benefit from the following supplements:

- Fiber supplements: If you don't get enough fiber from your diet, your doctor may offer a fiber supplement like psyllium husk or methylcellulose.

- Probiotic supplements: These can assist if you don't eat enough probiotic-rich foods or if you have a history of gastrointestinal issues.
- Other supplements: Some research suggests that certain supplements, like as fish oil or curcumin, may have anti-inflammatory qualities that can help patients with diverticulitis. However, further research is required in this field.

It is critical to check your doctor before beginning any new supplements, as they may conflict with specific drugs or not be suitable for everyone.

Remember:

- A fiber-rich diet is essential for long-term diverticulitis therapy.
- Consume a variety of fiber-rich foods in your diet.
- Consider using probiotics and prebiotics to improve gut health.
- Discuss any supplements with your doctor before starting them.

By making these dietary changes, you can take proactive actions to avoid future flare-ups and promote long-term digestive health.

<u>Lifestyle Changes for Prevention</u>

While dietary adjustments are important in preventing diverticulitis flare-ups, maintaining a healthy lifestyle is also essential.

The following lifestyle changes can help minimize your risk and boost general well-being:

Regular Exercise.

Regular physical activity provides numerous benefits for digestive health and diverticulitis prevention.

- Improved intestinal motility: Exercise stimulates the muscles in your intestines, encouraging regular bowel movements and reducing constipation, which is a major risk factor for diverticulitis.
- Weight management: Maintaining a healthy weight relieves pressure on your colon and reduces the likelihood of diverticula formation.
- Stress reduction: Physical activity can help manage stress, which is thought to be a trigger for flare-ups in certain people.

- Overall health benefits: Exercise helps your immune system, cardiovascular health, and mood, all of which lead to a healthier gut.

Most days of the week, aim to do at least 30 minutes of moderate-intensity activity, such as brisk walking, cycling, or swimming.

If you're new to exercising, begin slowly and gradually increase the duration and intensity over time.

Stress Reduction

Stress has a detrimental impact on your digestive system and may cause diverticulitis flare-ups. Implementing stress management practices will help you cope with life's problems while also promoting intestinal health.

Consider implementing the following stress-reduction techniques into your routine.

- Mindfulness and meditation: These activities can help you develop a sense of calm and focus, lowering anxiety and increasing relaxation.
- Yoga and tai chi are mild forms of exercise that blend movement, breath control, and meditation to promote both physical and mental health.

- Deep breathing exercises: Simple deep breathing methods can be conducted anywhere and at any time to promote relaxation and reduce tension.
- Spending time in nature: Studies have shown that connecting with nature reduces stress and improves mood.
- Participating in hobbies and activities you enjoy: Doing things you enjoy can provide a healthy distraction from tensions while also improving your general well-being.

Weight Management

Maintaining a healthy weight is critical to diverticulitis prevention. Excess weight puts strain on your colon, increasing the likelihood of diverticula formation and inflammation.

If you are overweight or obese, consult your doctor to design a safe and successful weight loss plan. This could include a combination of dietary adjustments, increased physical activity, and behavioral improvements.

Avoid Smoking and Excessive Alcohol Consumption.

- Smoking: It weakens the immune system, reduces blood flow, and raises the risk of a variety of health issues, including diverticulitis. Quitting smoking is one of the most beneficial things you can do for your overall health and digestive function.
- Excessive alcohol consumption might irritate the gut lining, increasing the risk of diverticulitis flare-ups. If you decide to drink alcohol, do so in moderation.

By making these lifestyle changes, you can take a proactive approach to avoiding diverticulitis flare-ups and improving long-term digestive health.

<u>**Regular Check-Ups and Monitoring.**</u>

While maintaining a healthy lifestyle and eating habits is critical for controlling diverticulitis, regular check-ups and monitoring with your healthcare practitioner are also essential for long-term health.

The importance of follow-up appointments

- Monitoring illness progression: Regular visits enable your doctor to evaluate the efficacy of your current treatment plan and make any required changes.
- Monitoring for complications: Even with good management, problems might occur. Regular check-ups enable early detection and management for any potential problems.
- Addressing any issues: This is an opportunity to bring up any new symptoms, questions, or concerns you may have regarding your health or treatment.

The frequency of follow-up appointments will be determined by your specific circumstances, the severity of your diverticulitis, and any other health concerns you may have.

Your doctor will provide particular recommendations based on your needs.

Addressing Concerns

Open contact with your healthcare physician is vital for successful diverticulitis treatment. Please do not hesitate to:

- Ask questions: If you have any questions or concerns about your illness, treatment options, or lifestyle suggestions, don't be reluctant to consult your doctor.
- Report new or worsening symptoms: Tell your doctor right away if you notice any new or worsening symptoms, no matter how small they appear.
- Discuss any difficulties: If you are having trouble adhering to dietary or lifestyle advice, consult your doctor. They can offer assistance and guidance to help you overcome any challenges.

By actively participating in your healthcare and maintaining open communication with your doctor, you can assure excellent diverticulitis therapy and reduce the risk of complications.

CHAPTER FIVE: LIVING WITH DIVERTICULITIS.

Coping With the Emotional Impact

Living with diverticulitis can be emotionally difficult, especially when flare-ups occur or the possibility of problems arises.

Recognizing and addressing these emotional aspects is critical for maintaining general well-being and navigating the path with resilience.

Understanding Emotional Challenges.

Diverticulitis can cause a variety of emotional responses, including:

- Anxiety and worry: The unpredictable nature of flare-ups, as well as the possibility of consequences, can cause anxiety and fear, interfering with everyday activities and decision-making.
- Irritation and fury: Dealing with persistent symptoms, food restrictions, and lifestyle changes can cause irritation and resentment.

- Depression and sadness: Physical restrictions and their impact on quality of life can cause feelings of melancholy and depression.
- Social isolation: Anxiety over controlling symptoms in social situations or while traveling can lead to avoidance and withdrawal.

It's crucial to realize that these feelings are natural and understandable. Recognizing and recognizing these emotions is the first step toward properly dealing with them.

Seeking Support.

You do not have to confront these issues alone. Seeking help from others can significantly improve your emotional well-being.

- Communicate with your loved ones: Discuss your sentiments and concerns with your family and friends. Their understanding and support can be really beneficial.
- Join a support group: Connecting with people going through similar experiences helps foster a sense of community and understanding. You can share information, offer encouragement, and learn coping skills from each other.

- Seek professional help: If you're having trouble coping with the emotional effects of diverticulitis, consider speaking with a therapist or counselor. They can provide tools and strategies for dealing with anxiety, sadness, and other emotional issues.

Remember:

- It is natural to have a variety of emotions when living with diverticulitis.
- Don't be afraid to seek help from loved ones, support groups, or mental health specialists.
- Integrate stress management practices into your daily routine to improve emotional well-being.

Maintaining A Positive Outlook.

While living with diverticulitis offers obstacles, maintaining a good attitude can have a big impact on your general well-being and capacity to manage the condition effectively.

Focus on Controllable Factors

Dealing with a chronic ailment like diverticulitis might make you feel overwhelmed or disappointed.

However, focusing on the things over which you have control can strengthen you and give you a sense of agency. This includes:

- Dietary choices: Eating a high-fiber diet and making intelligent food choices can greatly minimize the likelihood of flare-ups while also improving gut health.
- Lifestyle habits: Regular exercise, stress management strategies, and proper sleep can all help to improve general health and lower the risk of problems.
- Proactive self-care: Knowing your condition, getting regular check-ups, and communicating openly with your healthcare practitioner allow you to play an active part in your health.

By concentrating on these controllable aspects, you can change your perspective from feeling like a victim of your condition to feeling like an active participant in your own health journey.

Setting Goals and Celebrating Achievement

Setting realistic objectives and acknowledging your accomplishments, no matter how minor, can help you stay motivated and optimistic.

- Set SMART goals that are specific, measurable, attainable, relevant, and time-bound. Instead of saying "I want to eat healthier," make a goal like "I will incorporate two servings of vegetables into my lunch and dinner every day for the next week."
- Keep a notebook or use a tracking tool to track your progress toward your objectives. This might help you stay on track and envision your accomplishments.
- Celebrate your accomplishments: Recognize and reward yourself for meeting your objectives. This positive reinforcement might help you gain confidence and motivation.

Progress isn't always linear. There could be difficulties along the road. Be gentle with yourself, learn from any obstacles, and keep moving forward.

CHAPTER SIX: BONUS.

<u>Frequently Asked Questions.</u>

Common Concerns and Misconceptions.

Living with diverticulitis frequently prompts numerous questions and concerns.

This section answers some of the most frequently asked questions and dispels common misconceptions regarding the disease.

- Can I avoid diverticulitis entirely? While there is no 100% certain approach to avoid diverticulitis, eating a high-fiber diet, maintaining a healthy weight, exercising regularly, and quitting smoking can all help to minimize your risk.
- Is diverticulitis identical to colon cancer? No, diverticulitis and colon cancer are two separate conditions. However, certain symptoms may overlap, so visit your doctor for a full diagnosis and examination.
- Can I have nuts and seeds if I have diverticulitis? Historically, it was thought that nuts and seeds might

become lodged in diverticula and cause flare-ups. However, new evidence suggests that they are generally harmless for persons with diverticulitis and may even be advantageous when combined with a high-fiber diet.

- Will I require surgery for diverticulitis? Diverticulitis treatment does not necessarily require surgery. Many cases can be successfully controlled with conservative treatment, such as dietary adjustments, antibiotics, and pain relief. Recurrent flare-ups, complications, or severe symptoms, on the other hand, may warrant surgical intervention.

- Does stress cause diverticulitis? While stress does not directly cause diverticulitis, it can exacerbate flare-ups in some people. Managing stress with relaxation techniques and healthy lifestyle choices is critical for general well-being and digestion.

- Is diverticulitis hereditary? There could be a genetic tendency to diverticulosis and diverticulitis. If you have a family history of the condition, you should be aware of your risk and take precautions.

Expert Answers

In this part, we'll provide expert responses to some of the more specific questions that people with diverticulitis may have.

These answers are based on current medical knowledge and research, but it is always best to visit your doctor for specific guidance.

- Can I have popcorn if I have diverticulitis? Popcorn is typically not suggested during a flare-up since it is difficult to digest and may irritate the irritated colon. However, if your symptoms have eased, you can gradually resume consuming popcorn in moderation as part of a high-fiber diet.
- Which activity is best for diverticulitis? Any moderate-intensity activity that you love and can do on a regular basis is excellent for diverticulitis. Brisk walking, swimming, cycling, and yoga are all excellent choices.
- Does diverticulitis cause weight loss? Yes, diverticulitis can sometimes cause weight loss, especially during flare-ups. This could be related to a decrease in appetite, nausea, vomiting, or dietary restrictions. However, unintended weight loss should always be

investigated by a doctor to rule out any other underlying causes.

- Does diverticulitis effect fertility? Diverticulitis does not directly impair fertility. However, in rare situations, severe complications such as abscesses or fistulas can damage reproductive organs and impair fertility.
- Can diverticulitis be cured? While there is no cure for diverticulosis, the underlying illness that can cause diverticulitis, flare-ups can be effectively treated with the right therapy and lifestyle changes. By taking proactive actions to preserve gut health and avoid complications, you can reduce the impact of diverticulitis on your life.

This section seeks to answer common diverticulitis-related queries and misconceptions. However, it does not replace professional medical advice.

Always visit your doctor for personalized advice and answers to any particular inquiries you may have regarding your health.

CONCLUSION

Throughout this handbook, we've been on a quest to comprehend, manage, and eventually flourish after diverticulitis. We investigated the complexities of the ailment, its symptoms, and the many treatment choices available.

We've looked into the effectiveness of dietary and lifestyle changes, emphasizing the value of a high-fiber diet, frequent exercise, stress management, and proactive self-care.

Remember the following crucial points:

- Diverticulitis is a prevalent yet treatable illness.
- Early diagnosis and treatment are critical to avoiding problems.
- A high-fiber diet provides the foundation for long-term management.
- Lifestyle changes, such as exercise and stress reduction, are important in preventing disease and improving general health.
- Don't be afraid to seek help from loved ones, support groups, or mental health specialists.
- Maintain a good attitude and concentrate on the areas of your health that you can manage.

With the knowledge and tactics given in this manual, you can take control of your digestive health and confidently handle the obstacles of diverticulitis.

Remember, you are not alone on this path. Despite their illness, millions of people around the world have fulfilling lives.

We respect your input and would be delighted to hear about your experience with "The Ultimate Diverticulitis Handbook." Please take a time to provide an honest review and tell us how this book has helped you on your quest to digestive wellness. Your insights can inspire and empower others dealing with diverticulitis.

Remember that you are capable, resilient, and deserve a fulfilling life. Accept the knowledge you've received, take proactive efforts to improve your health, and continue to thrive after diverticulitis.